FROM WITCHCRAFT TO CHEMOTHERAPY

CAMBRIDGE
UNIVERSITY PRESS

University Printing House, Cambridge CB2 8BS, United Kingdom

Published in the United States of America by Cambridge University Press, New York

Cambridge University Press is part of the University of Cambridge.

It furthers the University's mission by disseminating knowledge in the pursuit of education, learning and research at the highest international levels of excellence.

www.cambridge.org
Information on this title: www.cambridge.org/9781107632455

© Cambridge University Press 1941

First published 1941
Re-issued 2014

A catalogue record for this publication is available from the British Library

ISBN 978-1-107-63245-5 Paperback

FROM WITCHCRAFT TO CHEMOTHERAPY

BY

SIR WALTER LANGDON-BROWN

*Emeritus Professor of Physic and Fellow of Corpus Christi College
in the University of Cambridge*

THE LINACRE LECTURE 1941

CAMBRIDGE

AT THE UNIVERSITY PRESS

1941

Magistro et Sociis
Coll. S. Johannis Evangelistae
grato animo
alumnus

FROM WITCHCRAFT TO
CHEMOTHERAPY

✼

IT is my pleasing duty in the first place to express my sincere thanks to the Master and Fellows of St John's College for the honour they have conferred on me by the invitation to deliver a lecture of such ancient tradition. They could have chosen others more worthy, but no one who could appreciate that distinction more. Thereby they have added still further to the great debt I owe the College. It is a responsible task which falls to my lot, that of carrying on a tradition despite all the alarums and excursions that beset us to-day. Jung must have been prophetically inspired when at Vienna in 1932 (note the date) he said: 'Once tradition has been sufficiently lopped off by...revolutionary unhistorical and therefore uneducated inclinations...leadership is the more fanatically defended the more unsuitable it is.' I think the twentieth century was born with a desire to cast aside the traditions of the nineteenth; every poet, sculptor, painter and musician loudly proclaimed that creed. Yet the results do not appear to have been particularly encouraging. The difficulty has always been to distinguish between a living tradition which can be modified to meet changing conditions and a dead one which cumbers the ground, obstructing growth. It is part of my purpose to-day to discuss the influence of some of the conflicts concerning traditions on thought and conduct.

The Influence of Tradition

Here at the very outset St John's College provides me with an illustration. The mediaeval universities as we know were not founded but just grew out of a sudden passionate desire for learning that was born with the twelfth century. Now it happened that the Hospital of St John had been founded in 1135 for a community of Augustinian Canons before university, hostel or college was in existence. Later Hugh de Balsham, who had become Bishop of

Ely in 1257, introduced into this hospital a certain number of the scholars who since the invitation of Henry III had been flocking to the University. Here he hoped they would be better cared for, but unfortunately the brethren and the scholars quarrelled incessantly. The original versions of Aristotle set free from Constantinople in 1204 were exciting profound interest everywhere and had given impetus to a new form of learning; the old and the new were incompatible, and, as has happened repeatedly, the old won. Balsham founded Peterhouse instead and the quarrelsome monks lost for my first college the distinction of being the oldest. The hospital clinging to the old tradition deteriorated so much that it was finally dissolved in 1510, only to arise again phoenix-like a year later as St John's College.

Another and more serious consequence of the conflict between old and new ideas is also associated with this College and this Lectureship, when Thomas Linacre, who had stimulated Henry VIII to found the Royal College of Physicians in 1518, himself founded lectureships, both here and at Oxford, in 1526. In 1540 this was followed by the establishment of the Regius Professorships. With these advantages it is disappointing to find how little was achieved. My distinguished predecessor in this lectureship, Professor Topley, had no hesitation in explaining this. He must have startled his audience when he said the only reason Linacre did no more harm than he did as a physician was because the times were too much for him, that his was the high tragedy of the wrong thing supremely well done, 'for he believed that the resurrection of the Greek physician in his pristine purity would put medicine on the right road again'. This is to be wise after the event, but it is true that Linacre was not interested in new observations; for him the *re*-naissance was literally to be a rebirth of the old culture. His whole outlook was authoritarian. The letter had been rediscovered but the spirit continued to elude him. Hence the comparative sterility of his benefactions for many years. Caius seems to me to have imbibed more of the new spirit from Padua than did

Linacre, and he introduced the practice of dissection at his College, where Harvey's interest in the subject of anatomy was presumably first aroused. He also initiated a new tradition by his treatise on the sweating sickness; a work based on direct clinical observation and not a mere quoting of authorities. Later in life, however, Caius became alarmed at the excesses which followed the exhilarating intoxication of the Renaissance and he began to wonder whether he had not done harm in encouraging the movement by his benefactions. In spite of his great services to medicine he seems to have died a disillusioned old man.

Linacre and Caius each founded institutions which have survived them to this day, yet they stand for two different reactions to the Renaissance; the former's robust belief in the mere restoration of the old seriously interfered with the efficacy of his gifts; the latter welcomed the new until its kaleidoscopic effect on religion and morals made him withdraw into his shell. But is this not the history of all new births? The excesses and terrors of the French Revolution made Edmund Burke aghast, while they changed Wordsworth from a revolutionary into a reactionary. When the crisis comes men fall into two groups, some look back and like Lot's wife become pillars of salt, the symbol of unavailing tears, while others look forward, determined that, at whatever cost, a new and better order shall arise out of chaos. Never was that faith more needed than to-day and, surely, never was it more difficult to cling to it.

This is to anticipate however, and we must return to the dawn of the seventeenth century, which saw the introduction of the method of experiment. Here for the third time St John's College comes into my story when John Gilbert, the third Johnian in direct succession to become President of the Royal College of Physicians, published his great treatise on the magnet and terrestrial magnetism, in 1600, the first book on physics with a modern outlook. Sir William Hale-White makes out a good case for the influence of this work on William Harvey, whose experiments had such far-reaching consequences.

Harvey's scientific attitude was not confined to the circulation or to embryology for, though it is perhaps less known, he applied it to his investigations on witchcraft, which were marked by humanity tempered by scepticism. And thus I reach my main topic—the origin of witchcraft from primitive religion and the part it played in the evolution of remedies through the magical phase to empirical success aided by laboratory investigation. Indeed the Greek word φαρμακεία originally meant a form of witchcraft; medicated drugs magically despatched to procure the death of misliked persons.

Religion and Magic

We realize now that myths and legends are not merely idle tales. Study of primitive people and especially Freud's technique for exploring the unconscious mind have taught us that legends represent history distorted by imagination, while myths embody men's hopes and fears, particularly fears. And so we are more prepared to listen to old wives' tales and try to assess their significance.

To do this we must go a long way back. Primaeval man found himself in a world that was hard to understand. Some things were predictable: the sequence of day and night, the phases of the moon, the succession of the seasons. But some things were not predictable, such as thunderstorms, floods and death. He felt himself at the mercy of unseen powers, and he desired to placate them. It is a testimony to the antiquity of the medical profession that the first individual to raise his head above the common herd was the medicine-man, who claimed and indeed acquired superior knowledge. As he frequently professed to justify the ways of God to man, his functions were generally blended with those of the priest. Among primitive people all disease is regarded as coming from without by evil influences, human or divine. Therefore it seemed to them that effective remedies could only be provided by magic. Now magic assumed three main forms—sympathetic magic which reappeared in semi-scientific form in the homœopathic dictum 'like cures like', contagious magic, the forerunner of plasters and poultices, and incantations of which hypnosis may be regarded as the modern equivalent. It is not surprising that since magic was relied upon for so many centuries, there is still a craving for magical cures. Is not the highest praise we can give to a remedy that it worked like magic? And how many of you can lay your hand on your heart and swear that you never touch wood to avert disaster, never throw spilled salt over your left shoulder, never bow to the new moon or try to avoid the number 13?

Primitive man was animistic, endowing everything with a spirit. Beside the great gods there were innumerable local spirits—every stream and fountain had its nymph, every tree its dryad, every hillside its oread. As tribes began to mingle, their myths began to fuse. It was recognized that the fertility of the land depended on two things, the sun's rays and the nymph-haunted waters. There was only one sun, and many rivers. Therefore when the local myths fused, the fertile land had one father but many mothers. Hence Jupiter was saddled with a highly polygamous character, and one which has unfairly stuck to him.

We shall find these gods of the soil, chthonic deities as they were called, are of great importance to our present subject, for from them sprang the idea of herbal magic. When man began to settle down to cultivate the soil, he became impressed with the importance of private ownership. He set up boundary stones —and 'cursed be he who removeth his neighbour's landmark'. These stones thus acquired special sanctity. When Jacob and Laban quarrelled about their property they set up a boundary pillar, calling it Mizpah as a witness to their pact against aggression into the other's territory; not quite the same idea that impels lovers to have Mizpah engraved inside an engagement ring! Thus the boundary stone becomes a god, and before long a face is carved upon it—the terminal figure with which it is still customary to decorate gardens as if to guard them against marauders.

Such crude conceptions of deity could not continue to satisfy man's feelings. Thus in

Greek mythology the Term or Herm (the names were interchangeable) became Hermes, or for the Romans, Mercury, who rising from the ground took to himself winged cap and sandals to become the swift messenger of the sky gods on snowy Olympus. Even to-day he serves the modern gods of speed and advertisement, 'Oh Mr Mercury you *did* give me a start.' It was all very well to have a terminal god to guard your territory, but unless that land produced good crops it was not much use to you. A plentiful harvest was one of the unpredictable things. If it had not been for submarines it would never have occurred to us that a bad harvest might spell starvation; yet it was not until well on in the eighteenth century that import of grain from overseas made us practically independent of bad harvests in this country. Imagine what they must have meant for small communities surrounded by hostile tribes. No wonder that seed time and harvest were times of anxiety and excitement; and that the gods were called upon for aid, and thanked when the earth was generous—a custom which survives in the Church to-day in the Harvest Festival. The whole of Greek Drama was evolved from ritual dances that took place round the threshing floor during these phases of excitement. To this day ritual dances are performed before the high altar in Seville Cathedral at Easter to celebrate the resurrection. In other words the earliest form of organized religion was a fertility religion. H. G. Wells surmises that it was noticed that where the soil had been turned over to make a grave for a chief, corn grew more abundantly, and this led to the well-known idea that there must be a human sacrifice to ensure a good crop. The better the victim the better the crop —he was, as it were, a sacrificial god-king. And Wells goes on to visualize a scene at Avebury: 'Away beyond the dawn of history 3,000 or 4,000 years ago, one thinks of the Wiltshire uplands in the twilight of a mid-summer's day morning. The torches pale in the growing light. One has a dim apprehension of a procession through the avenue of stone, of priests fantastically dressed...of chiefs...

bearing spears and axes...of a great peering crowd of shock-headed men and naked children....A certain festive cheerfulness prevails. And amid the throng march the appointed human victims, submissive, helpless, staring towards the distant smoking altar at which they are to die—that the harvests may be good and the tribe increase.' And as I re-read that passage I recalled the long succession of bonfires on Midsummer Eve I saw last year in the Irish countryside hungrily crackling; but the sacrificial victims were elsewhere.

When Christianity replaced the old nature-worship these fires were not abruptly interdicted, but their significance was adroitly changed. Of old their kindling was to ensure the continuance of plant-life; now they did honour to St John and his martyrdom, which blessed the plants that bloomed in that season of the year. On St John's Eve the spirits of the dead had leave to wander on earth for a few hours, and 'when at midnight the hooting of an owl in the woods or a rustle of a sparrow in the ivy portended the presence of the souls of the dead, the trembling doctor, alone and in silence, went out to pull the herbs of grace'. Culled otherwise they would have no medicinal virtue.

At a certain stage in human development the better minds in a community begin to revolt against a mere fertility religion and to find refuge in a mystery religion. I shall only take an example of this, the Eleusinian Mysteries of ancient Greece. It is a wonderful experience to drive down between the hills, clothed in olive groves, past the lovely little Byzantine Convent of Daphni with its glowing mosaics to the bay of Salamis on the shores of which lie the ruins of the great temples of Eleusis. Here for centuries youths from all over the then civilized world went to undergo as it were a second birth, an initiation into adult life. After a sojourn in a dark cave they were brought up into a brilliantly lighted hall. Carved reliefs that were found there tell us something of the imagery by which they were instructed. We see Persephone or Proserpine rising from the ground to renew the flowers, and Demeter or

«(18)»

Ceres handing to the youth some ears of corn, while in the background is a man holding the torch of life. From the flowers and the corn the young men were taught concerning the handing on of human life, and led up to a conception of a divine principle in man and woman. Finally, the hope of a personal immortality was held out for the first time in the Greek world. St Paul spoke the very language of the Eleusinian mysteries in that famous passage beginning 'Except a corn of wheat fall into the ground and die', a passage fraught to this day with poignant associations. That the influence of Eleusis was for good there is abundant evidence from classical literature. It is in accord with the less pleasing aspects of human nature that on their return to Athens the initiated were received with ribald jests. Man takes a curious pleasure in smearing divine mysteries with a clumsy thumb—witness to-day the boorish speeding of the newly married couple on their honeymoon.

The third stage in an organized religion is to emphasize the spiritual side and to repress its overt association with fertility rites. The Greeks symbolized this by the gradual elevation of the earth gods to the heights of Olympus. Perhaps spiritual is too strong a word to apply to Greek religion—it was rather the elevation of the rational intellectual spirit over the instinctive fears of primitive man. It has always been a great difficulty for man to harmonize these different sides of his nature. The ascetic path is a denial of the instinctive levels, but it is one fraught with some real dangers. See how again and again the Israelites returned to their fertility rites—the worship of the golden calf, the worship of Baal and Ashtaroth and the sacred groves that Josiah cut down. Saul bewildered and outwitted by the wily Samuel reverts and consults the witch of Endor. Do we not see the same thing in our Gothic cathedrals? The soaring arches and the rose windows draw our eyes heavenwards, but look under the miserere seats in the choir stalls and you see grotesque carvings of fables and of human weaknesses. In Paris the towers of Notre-Dame point to the skies, but on its terraces are strange inhuman monsters, while a goblin-like figure leans over the parapet with outstretched tongue, leering balefully at the city below. To-day he must be jeering at the ways of man more than ever as he watches captured Caliban taking Ariel captive again.

Witchcraft and Fairies

Thus, if we are to comprehend witchcraft we must see it as an expression of the thwarted instinctive self turned renegade and forcing its way into consciousness again with an evil leer. Witchcraft and fertility rites had seized on the imagination of people thousands of years before the introduction of Christianity. Indeed the oldest representation of a god is the Stag Man or Hooded God painted on the walls of a cave at Ariège, 8,000 years ago during the old Stone Age. Down through the ages he roams, posing as Pan in Greece, as Herne the Hunter in Windsor Forest, and still reappears to this day in the Horn Dance in Shropshire, as well as in the ballet based on Berlioz's 'Symphonie Fantastique'.

Too often the tales of wholesale conversions of races to Christianity must be regarded as merely synonymous with conquest. Pagan tribes 'were pitchforked into the Christian fold at the point of the sword, straight from the level of polydaemonism and nature worship into a mystical Eastern religion, with which their own indigenous myth had nothing in common' (H. G. Baynes). It is not surprising therefore that just as the Israelites of old frequently relapsed, so did masses of the British people revert to their ancient rites, though their rulers professed Christianity. Dr Margaret Murray has given a fascinating account of this, which I will attempt to paraphrase. It is only to be expected that it was among the older races oppressed by the invaders that these ancient cults would persist most firmly. Now the skeletal remains in the Neolithic burial barrows show that they were a short race—the men about 5 feet 5 inches and the women proportionately less. Hence the name of 'The Little People'; and it is interesting to note that many of the witch-beliefs and practices coincide with those of an existing dwarf race, the Lapps. Later the 'little people' were called fairies. Outcast and outlawed they dwelt in forests or on the hills, whence they descended to raid the flocks. It was from our ancestors of the Iron Age (i.e. about 1,000 B.C.) that the traditional fear of the fairies was derived, the terror of the implacable enemy, who, having only flint weapons to match against metal ones, had to win by cunning and stratagem. To this day in parts of the country the flint arrow-heads are called elf-arrows. Belonging to the 'little people' is Robin Hood, really Robin with a hood, i.e. the hooded stag man; he is a legendary figure widely spread in place and time. He was always accompanied by a band of 12, which we shall see was significant. He wore the fairy's colour, green—no doubt for protective camouflage, whether hunter or hunted. In all the stories his animosity to the Church is stressed and an Abbot or a Prior was regarded as his legitimate prey; naturally so, since he was the totem of the opposing cult. Of the same order was Robin Goodfellow or Puck, that

'Lob of spirits' recently reincarnated by Barrie in *Dear Brutus*. In some parts of the country women dislike wearing green dresses because they believe the next dress will be black for mourning. Is this the lingering of an old idea that the fairies will punish anyone who steals their colour?

It is not too much to say that the authentic fairies, as described here, died in the Black Death. Dr Murray amusingly says they were eaten by the sheep, and this is how it came about. The terrible scarcity of labour after that devastating pestilence led to development of sheep farming for the wool merchant, sheep requiring fewer men. It was the stapling and weaving of wool which restored prosperity to the land, and wherever that industry prevailed we still find beautiful villages, such as Lavenham in East Anglia and Chipping Campden in the west country, indicating the wealth of the district. Now we must observe that in grazing the difference between cattle and sheep is very marked—for cattle the grass must be sufficiently long for the animal to put its tongue round a bunch of grass and break it off—the grass which is left is not bitten down to the roots. By the formation of their teeth sheep are able to nibble the grass almost to the roots. Thus sheep can graze after cattle but not cattle after sheep. Sheep can also find a living on ground which cannot support cattle. As these 'fairies' were cattle keepers the advent of the sheep must have driven them out of their old haunts. There would be no feed for their beasts as in the old days. The real upland dwellers who struck terror into the lowlanders and horrified the priests of Christian faith vanished utterly.

The present conception of fairies is due to Shakespeare. The ancient Greek writers calmed the fears of the people by converting their obsessional alarms into beautiful myths, although, as Mr G. M. Young has recently pointed out, there are vestiges of primitive totemism in Aeschylus. Shakespeare did the same by turning Puck into the service of Oberon, and 'debunking' the terrors of Herne the Hunter by dressing up Falstaff as such, but most of all by making the 'little people' still more minute. People couldn't be frightened by anything so tiny as Mercutio's Queen Mab, or as Pease Blossom. When Granville-Barker produced *A Midsummer-Night's Dream* he claimed that he was correct in representing fairies as full-sized men. But in doing this he was taking a pre-Shakespearian view. Nevertheless, it must be admitted that in *The Merry Wives of Windsor* Anne Page not only dressed up as a fairy but expected to be taken as such, though a full-grown young woman. But here as in *A Midsummer-Night's Dream* the whole fairy atmosphere is playful. I take Shakespeare's object to have been to strip the countryside of bogies and 'things that go bump in the night' and to show that the real terrors are the conflicts within the human soul.

Historically it appears clear that witchcraft was the persistent vestige of the old fertility religion. The devotees formed themselves into 'covens' of 12, making with their leader the ominous number 13. Dr Murray shows that there was a close association between our highest order of knighthood and these rites.

A special garter was often worn as the emblem of belonging to the Old Religion. The foundation of the Order of the Garter after the Countess of Salisbury dropped hers while dancing with Edward III suggests that her confusion was not from a shock to her modesty —it took more than that to shock a lady of the fourteenth century—but the possession of that garter proved that she was not only a member of the Old Religion but held the highest place in it. She therefore stood in imminent danger from the Church, which had already started on its career of persecution. The King's quickness in making it the insignia for himself placed him at the head of the Old Religion also in the eyes of his pagan subjects. It is noteworthy that he followed this up by the foundation of an order of 12 knights for the King and 12 for the Prince of Wales, i.e. 2 covens. Curiously enough the riband of the Order of the Garter is blue, whereas that of the fertility rites was green, as exemplified in the folk-dance known as Green Garters which carried the procession to the May Pole and was throughout England the customary introduction to the May Pole rites. Note also the old custom of the struggle for the bride's garters, now fallen into deserved desuetude. Herrick, for instance, in his verses on the marriage of his friend Sir Clipsby Crew adjures the bride to

Let the young-men and the Bride-maids share
　　　　Your garters.

I had the pleasure of calling Dr Murray's attention to the scene at Herne's Oak in the *Merry Wives* which conclusively proves the correctness of her view, where Sweet Anne Page in fairy attire addresses her fellow sprites thus:

And nightly, meadow-fairies, look you sing,
Like to the Garter's compass, in a ring:
The expressure that it bears, green let it be,
More fertile-fresh than all the field to see;
And 'Honi soit qui mal y pense' write
In emerald tufts, flowers purple, blue, and white;
Like sapphire, pearl and rich embroidery,
Buckled below fair knighthood's bending knee:
Fairies use flowers for their charactery.
Away; disperse; but till 'tis one o'clock,
Our dance of custom round about the oak
Of Herne the hunter, let us not forget.

Indeed the whole scene is packed with folk-lore, and amid delightful confusion Herne the Hunter is attacked by the fairies themselves, who inflict their customary pinchings and burning on that object of fear, the Stag-God. Revealed as only that absurd Falstaff after all, the myth is killed by ridicule. Fear is banished by laughter.

De Lancre, writing in 1662, said: 'There are two sorts of witches, one who gave themselves up to drugs and poison, the others perform wonders.' We are concerned with the former, but it is of interest to deal here with the old wives' tale of witches riding on broom-sticks, because we shall find it concerns both aspects of witchcraft. In mediaeval representations of ritual witch dances the women hold brooms and the men pitchforks, the broom thus becoming regarded as a feminine symbol. The original broom, whether for domestic or magical purposes, was a stalk of the broom plant with a tuft of leaves at the end. The plant was believed to have magical qualities, particularly in the giving or blasting of fertility.

Note the old gipsy marriage rite of jumping over the broom-stick and an old saying in some parts of England, 'If you sweep the house with blossomed broom in May you sweep the head of the house away.' Yet as far as we know the only action of the scoparium, which broom yields, is that of a mild diuretic. More interesting is the composition of the flying ointments that witches employed in their attempts to anticipate the aeroplane as a harbinger of evil. My friend Professor A. J. Clark, examining the recipes for such ointments, shows that aconite and belladonna are among the ingredients; the former would produce irregular action of the heart and the latter would cause delirium. 'Irregular action of the heart in a person falling asleep produces the well-known sensation of suddenly falling through space and it seems quite possible that the combination of a delirium-producing drug like belladonna with one producing irregular action of the heart like aconite might produce the sensation of flying.' He thinks that sooner or later the sensation of flying would be felt and the rider would be convinced that she had flown through the air. The usual attendant familiar on such flights of fancy was of course a black cat, and in remote parts of Ireland few of these animals are seen with intact tails, because from this mystic association their blood is believed to cure erysipelas, shingles and various other skin diseases. Hence these poor creatures have their tails nipped off bit by bit to perform the cure.

Witchcraft died out sooner in England than in Scotland, simply because it was persecuted less, for nothing stimulates a religion more than persecution. Yet it is estimated that something like two million persons were burned as witches throughout Europe in the space of a hundred years. To us it seems almost incredible that in the seventeenth century such men as Sir Thomas Browne, Henry More, and Joseph Glanvill should have believed in witches. But we must remember they felt that to doubt the existence of evil spirits implied an equal doubt in the existence of beneficent spiritual forces. In appealing to demonology, they were tapping a deep reservoir of traditional belief which could not be eradicated from the imagination despite the struggle towards higher levels of thought. 'For many, and in some cases subconscious motives men wished to believe in witchcraft'—and 'the intellect generally follows the emotions'. It was the peaceful penetration of the scientific outlook which ultimately destroyed the belief in witchcraft.

Folk-Lore in the Old Testament

And now let me refer to two curious instances of folk-lore in the Old Testament. When the Philistines captured the Ark of the Covenant and took it to Ashdod, 'there was a deadly destruction throughout all the city' by an epidemic. 'And the men that died not were smitten with the emerods: and the cry of the city went up to heaven.' So the Philistines called for the priests and the diviners to ask what trespass offering they should make to be healed. They answered: 'Five golden emerods and five golden mice.' Now the word 'emerod' is of course a corruption of the French word for haemorrhoid in which the 'h' would not be sounded. It has been pointed out, however, by scholars that the original Hebrew word might equally well mean bubo, i.e. the swollen inguinal glands of bubonic plague. That would explain the devastating mortality, which haemorrhoids certainly would not. Even the men of Bethshemesh who looked into the Ark on the return journey perished by thousands. Now I would like to call your special attention to the statement that it was the men who did not die who were smitten with emerods, for it is clearly recognized that in epidemics of plague the septicaemic and pneumonic forms are much more fatal than the cases accompanied by inguinal buboes. The trespass offering of golden mice particularly interests me. When there was a recurrence of plague in India in 1896 it was noted that when villagers saw a dead rat they quitted that village. Then at the Haffkine Institute it was shown that a human epidemic could be accurately foretold 2–3 weeks beforehand from a rising curve of infection in the rat population. Ultimately the carrier was found to be the flea on the rat, which deserts it on the animal's death, and may then infect man by its bite. Other rodents are also susceptible, and so it appears possible that the diviners among the Philistines in some vague way associated mice with plague and offered up mice in golden effigy to invoke sympathetic magic. It suggests that the Philistines were not so barbarous as the Israelites made out.

The other instance relates to a charm which persisted into my student days, and for all I know may still persist. When I was doing 'midwifery on the district' we noted that the Gamp in attendance always tried to slip a pat of butter mixed with brown sugar into the new-born infant's mouth. We were told not to allow this, but the *sage-femme* generally managed to outmanœuvre us! In the country the proper mixture is butter and honey, but if honey cannot be obtained brown sugar is substituted. They rationalize the procedure by saying it is good for the infant's bowels or some such story. I was delighted when I was reminded by Dr Murray that among the Messianic prophecies in the book of Isaiah is this: 'Butter and honey shall he eat, that he may know to refuse the evil and choose the good.' Evidently it was originally given as a charm and has lingered on as an assumed therapeutic measure. Is it not possible that originally the charm was intended to evade by homœopathic magic the primal threat in the Garden of Eden: 'But of the tree of the knowledge of good and evil thou shalt not eat: for in the day that thou eatest thereof thou shalt surely die.'

Herbal Remedies

I have attempted to show that the old wives' tales concerning magical cures are based on witchcraft which in its turn arose from the fertility cults. I will now briefly consider a few instances in which ancient folk-lore has led empirically to useful therapeutic discoveries. Really there are comparatively few recognized instances of this, considering the enormous prevalence of magical remedies employed throughout the ages. Yet Dr Dan Mackenzie gives 137 modern botanical remedies which undoubtedly emanated from folk-medicine, 25 that probably did, and 17 that possibly did. In addition he gives a list of 13 poisonous herbs recognized as such in folk-lore. Clearly it is only possible to allude to a few of the more striking examples.

Mandrake has been regarded as a magical plant from very remote ages and entered into the Druidical midsummer festivals. Some of the myths and superstitions arose from the real or fancied resemblance of mandrake to the human figure. When torn out of the ground it was believed to emit horrible shrieks. It was really a narcotic of considerable power, but was removed from the Pharmacopœia in 1746 and has never been replaced. It is probable that the superstitions connected with the mandrake were responsible for its rejection indirectly as well as directly, for we are told that in response to the enormous demand for mandrake by the later mediaeval physicians, the root of the bryony was faked up and sold instead of it; so that when our professional predecessors believed that they were using the potent root, they were, as a matter of fact, only handling an inert substitute. The Elizabethans regarded it in the same light as the poppy, as can be seen in Shakespeare's. *Othello*:

> Not poppy, nor mandragora,
> Nor all the drowsy syrups of the world
> Shall ever medicine thee to that sweet sleep....

The *poppy* was held by the Greeks to be sacred to Ceres, doubtless owing to its frequent appearance in corn fields. When Ceres was sorrowfully searching for her lost Proserpine she took no food but drank some poppy juice to secure rest. You are probably familiar with the beautiful bronze head of Hypnos, the God of Sleep, in the British Museum—with half-closed eyes and the wings of dreamland, one of them unfortunately broken. There is a much more perfect version in marble in the Prado Museum at Madrid, from which we can see that Hypnos was represented as a lovely youth carrying a wand in one hand and with the other squeezing a poppy over the sleeper. Of the opium the poppy yields it may truly be said that it is one of the greatest gifts of nature to man, and one which he often shamelessly misuses. In the Middle Ages the poppy like belladonna and hyoscyamus was esteemed to have been created by the devil for the benefit of witches, showing that its poisonous properties were clearly recognized. The older physicians were very chary of using *belladonna*, leaving it to witches, charlatans and poisoners, so that it fell into complete neglect and did not appear in the official list till 1832. *Hyoscyamus* prepared from henbane was not so much feared and was largely used by physicians in spite of its association with witchcraft. It was removed from the Pharmacopœia in 1746 but restored to the official list in 1809 after its properties had been scientifically examined.

The ancients were fully acquainted with the poisonous property of *aconite* from monks-hood. Medea prepared her deadly potions from it and it was also employed as an arrow poison. It was not employed in medicine, however, until 1762. *Conium* from hemlock was the poison that Socrates was condemned to drink. Plato's moving account of his death is a classic, describing how the coldness of his extremities gradually spread upwards till it reached his heart, though his mind remained clear to the end. Conium was the plant of Satan and the witches in folk-lore, but was not officially used till 1760; although still in the Codex it has now passed into complete disuse, though I remember Dr Samuel Gee prescribing succus conii for whooping cough. This raises an interesting point. Conium has a mouse-like odour, and roast or fried mouse is one of the earliest folk-lore remedies and has been used for whooping cough all over England. Did the similarity of the smell suggest this nasty remedy?

Cinchona is a drug we owe to Peruvian folk-lore and *mistletoe* has always had magical properties ascribed to it. According to Sir James Frazer this was because it was believed to have dropped on to the oak from the heavens in a flash of lightning, and in some parts of Switzerland mistletoe is still called thunder besom. Indeed he identified the Golden Bough with mistletoe seen through the haze of poetry and superstition. When the Druids cut mistletoe they always used a golden sickle and the branches were caught in a white sheet, never being allowed to have contact with the ground. It was used for epilepsy, often called the falling sickness, and I suspect the tale that it fell from the heavens suggested its employment as sympathetic magic. Nicholas Culpeper, that sturdy old herbalist who in 1652 wrote, 'As for the Colledg of Physitians they are too stately to learn and too proud to continue', had a great opinion of the virtues of mistletoe. He prescribed it not only for epilepsy but also for palsy and giddiness. Now each of those symptoms may occur from high blood pressure, and of recent years mistletoe has formed an ingredient of several remedies which are claimed to lower blood pressure.

Wormwood still figures in the Codex, though I imagine seldom prescribed, for its essential oil has rightly given absinthe a bad name; nevertheless it is contained in Vermouth and Chartreuse, and as it has a selective action on nerve centres its pharmaceutical effect might well be further investigated.

Chamomile is one of the few herbal remedies indigenous to England which was retained in the British Pharmacopœia till recently and still figures in the Codex, but its glories are those of a day that has gone, for its feeble qualities seldom lead to its being prescribed. All that is left of its former reputation as a panacea is that its flowers are used externally as a fomentation for bruises and contusions, though chamomile tea is still used as a domestic remedy.

Scurvy grass has an interesting bearing on our subject. Originally a folk-lore remedy for scurvy, it became official for a time and was then discarded. Now there is a very ancient tradition that children are liable to skin eruptions in the spring, just as plants burst into flower. Really such eruptions occur not because spring is beginning but because it is the end of winter when even now, but much more so in the past, the supply of vitamin C in the food is at its lowest ebb. Even fresh milk will contain less because the cows have eaten so little fresh vegetables. Now scurvy grass contains a pepper, and in quite recent years it has been shown that some peppers are rich in vitamin C. The Elizabethans were very keen on obtaining pepper fields, if necessary by force from other nations. They regarded pepper as a good food preservative—but it is more, it is an antiscorbutic. Only in little more than the last decade has the old wives' tale concerning scurvy grass received scientific sanction.

Digitalis (foxglove) was first given for consumption. The principal scientific writers were very generous in the number of diseases they treated with it, a circumstance which makes the absence of heart disease or dropsy from the list all the more striking. Withering in 1785 learned that foxglove was the main ingredient in an old secret family remedy for dropsy obscurely derived from ancient folk-medicine. In England it was looked upon as the fairy's plant par excellence, and inside its purple bells the elves were wont to hide when chased from their dances by the sound of a human foot. The witches, too, were fond of the plant and used to decorate their fingers with its flowers. Therefore it probably owes its introduction into medicine to magical thought.

Valerian is an interesting example of a useful drug that was originally employed as a love philtre. I cannot agree with Dr Ernest Jones when he says:

For a great many centuries asafoetida and valerian were administered on the grounds that hysteria was due to the wandering of the uterus about the body, and that evil-smelling drugs tended to drive it down to its proper position and thus cure the complaint. Although these assumptions have not been upheld by experience, nevertheless at the present day most cases of hysteria are still treated by these drugs. Evidently the operating influence that leads to their administration is the blind response to a prevailing tradition, the origin of which is largely forgotten. But the necessity of teachers of neurology to provide reasons to students for their treatment has led to the explanation being invented that the drugs act as 'antispasmodics'—whatever that may mean—and they are often given in the following refined form: One of the constituents of valerian—valerianic acid—is given the name of 'active principle', and is administered, usually as the zinc salt, sugar-coated so as to disguise its unpleasant taste. Some modern authorities, aware of the origin of the treatment, have even remarked how curious it is that the ancients, in spite of their false views about hysteria, should have discovered a valuable line of treatment and yet given such an absurd explanation of its action.

At the risk of being labelled a 'rationalizer' of effete superstitions, I venture to assert that I have never regarded the exhibition of valerian as a punitive measure. In fact, when patients need valerian they frequently do not appear to dislike it. The older observers often empirically determined the usefulness of a drug without understanding its mode of action—of this quinine is an historical example. The effect of valerian in a case of diabetes insipidus can be determined by direct observation, and is similar to that of amidopyrine and various hypnotics in this disease. Before the introduction of pituitrin in its treatment I had repeated opportunities of confirming this. Incidentally, Dr Ernest Jones, although an ardent Freudian, ignores the veiled symbolism which modern psychology has revived, though not in such a materialistic form, by attributing many hysterical symptoms to sexual causes.

The Evolution of Therapeutics

Herbal remedies and other crude methods lingered long in medicine because chemistry had not advanced sufficiently to form any basis for rational therapeutics. There was some excuse for herbalists in the days when the London Pharmacopœia for 1682 included the famous Theriaca of Mithridates, which contained some seventy ingredients. The eighteenth century being the Age of Reason was in no mood to continue such farragos, as Dr William Heberden contemptuously described them. Yet that eminent Johnian's own purge of the Pharmacopœia in 1746 was almost too drastic, and along with many useless preparations some valuable drugs were excluded, which have had to be reinstated subsequently. Indeed the therapeutics of that period and for many years later seem to have been devoted mainly to depressant methods such as salivation, emetics, purging and above all bleeding. When, by the

«(45)»

end of the eighteenth century, a new chemistry was beginning to appear, it naturally had its effect on pharmacology, and a number of empirical remedies were transformed into rational procedures. Nevertheless, a number of quite useless remedies continued to encumber the Pharmacopœia even up to the time when I unfortunately had to memorize them as a medical student. The more conservative members of the profession still held out against their deletion. I attribute the slow growth of therapeutics during the nineteenth century until its last decade to the fact that medicine then was so largely based on morbid anatomy. This emphasis on end results led to a spirit of nihilistic scepticism as to the value of drugs among many physicians. Looking at the extensive lesions then revealed, they were inclined to ask how could a bottle of medicine have prevented this, instead of concentrating on treatment before this stage was reached. Still, the sum total of reliable drugs slowly grew and the introduction of hypodermic medication by a great predecessor of mine in the Regius Chair,

Sir Clifford Allbutt, marked a new era in therapeutics.

The last decade of the nineteenth century was a great one in the history of medicine. Within five years the first endocrine was given, the first antitoxin injected, while X-rays and radium were discovered. This was shortly after an eminent authority had given his opinion that we had reached the end of great discoveries in medicine! A man would indeed have been gifted with prophetic vision if he could have realized then whither the first discovery of endocrines and antitoxins would lead. It may be said that the use of organic extracts was nothing new. Celsus and Galen testify to the antiquity of organo-therapy. But it was employed as a kind of sympathetic magic. The savage ate the heart of his adversary to obtain his courage, and powdered heart muscle was a favourite prescription in the old days; it is no advance to squeeze it into a tablet and call it cardin.

I must not take up your time by detailing the story of the birth of the new scientific organo-therapy which I heard from that distinguished Johnian, Professor G. R. Murray himself, who initiated it in 1891 by the successful use of thyroid extract in myxoedema.

The Natural and Acquired Defences of the Body

I need not enlarge on the triumphs of endocrine therapy, so powerfully aided by the hypodermic needle and the labours of the organic chemist. What I wish to point out is the new spirit of hopefulness it infused into therapeutics. Whenever we give a drug we imply thereby a belief that the functions of the body can be influenced by chemical means. New support for this confidence was found in the fact that the body itself produces chemical substances whereby it regulates its own functions. Nothing could be more reasonable than to use intelligently in disease those very drugs by which the body is enabled to do its own work in health. Thus we employ an endocrine in substitution therapy, or to diminish the action of its too exuberant opponent, or even simply for its pharmacological action. I am glad that

Professor Murray, always so modest and unassuming, lived long enough to see the acorn he planted, despite opposition, grow into a flourishing oak in whose shelter many have found relief and healing.

So much for the innate chemical defences of the body. The next step was the recognition of the way in which it could acquire new defences against attack, i.e. the antitoxins. The first of these and one of the most successful was diphtheria antitoxin introduced in 1894. It was realized that this merely conferred a passive immunity, and the next stage was to find ways in which active immunity could be acquired. Sir Almroth Wright was not to be deterred by the failures of others and in the closing years of the nineteenth century introduced the general conception of vaccines, adapting a word already well known to a principle already comprehended in theory. After forty years we have a fairly accurate idea both of the usefulness and limitations of this procedure, and I think it is fair to say that although it has by no means fulfilled all the early enthusiastic expectations, it has an undoubted field of usefulness. For myself I feel that it has been more successful as a prophylactic than as a cure. Certainly the statistics as to the value of inoculation against the typhoid group of infections in warfare are most impressive.

The next great advance arose from the recognition of deficiency diseases, the fact that a minus was as capable of producing a disease as a plus, so to speak. In Cambridge this aspect is so well known and so closely associated with the name of Sir Gowland Hopkins that I need not dilate upon it now. Suffice it to say that vitamins are all essential to some stage in the intimate biochemistry of the cell. Their scientific employment in therapeutics has been aided in some instances by methods which enabled the extent of their deficiency in an individual to be quantitatively estimated. Further, this work removed certain treatments such as whole rice for beri-beri, lemons for scurvy and cod-liver oil for rickets from the field of empiricism to that of rational therapeutics.

These triple discoveries of endocrines, antitoxins, whether actively or passively acquired, and vitamins have had a profound reaction on the whole subject of therapeutics, directing it towards the application of nature's own remedies. The next chapter, however, showed us how drugs foreign to the system could usefully intervene. When adrenaline was isolated and its pharmacological actions studied in detail, Langley pointed out in 1901 that these actions all resembled stimulation of the sympathetic nerves to any structure. The far-reaching significance of his generalization was not grasped for some twenty years. Then came the important researches of Dale and, independently, of Loewi. They found not only that adrenaline was liberated at every sympathetic terminal when its nerve was stimulated, but also that at every other type of nerve ending acetyl-cholin was momentarily set free. In other words all nervous impulses act on the tissues through the intermediary of chemical agents. It had long been known that atropin, for example, paralysed vagal and certain other nerve endings; now it was shown that this was because atropin prevented the access of the acetyl-cholin into the tissue cell. Conversely physostigmin was known to increase the effect of vagus stimulation; now it was shown that this was because the drug prevented the destruction of the acetyl-cholin by a special ferment and thus prolonged its action. Moreover, drugs may apparently prevent the entrance of toxin into the tissues. Thus G. N. Myers found that digitalis would prevent diphtheria toxin from getting into heart muscle. The adrenal medulla is just one large receptacle of the same chemical substance which is momentarily set free at every sympathetic post-ganglionic ending, and can reinforce the effects at such endings when there is a sudden emergency call for a general mobilization of the sympathetic nervous system.

Here we see a large field for pharmacological research and its therapeutical application opening out. Drugs can be used to facilitate or inhibit certain nervous reactions and to prevent toxic effects. Already synthetic modifications of acetyl-cholin such as mecholin have been shown to possess some but not all the properties of acetyl-cholin. Then the passage of normal acetyl-cholin into the muscles can be facilitated in myasthenia gravis by prostigmin, allied to natural physostigmin. The future seems full of promise for the development of such modifications. Particularly is this true of the synthetic endocrines, where Dodds has been able to indicate certain basal groups of simpler chemical structure than the natural endocrines which can act, as he phrases it, as pass-keys to the physiological lock.

We may well wonder how such powerful chemical substances circulating in the body exercise their action at the appropriate spot. Langley and also T. R. Elliot found it necessary to postulate the existence of an equally selective receptive substance in the tissue acted upon, and although we have as yet no notion of what such substances are, it is clear they exist. How otherwise can we account for the fact that thyroid extract will simultaneously speed up the atrophy of a tadpole's gills and the growth of its limbs? Or that injection of the pituitary growth hormone will still further elongate the already long backbone of a dachshund while it increases the length of a collie's legs? Evidently the success or failure of these natural drugs depends on some innate or acquired capacity of the individual to respond.

Chemotherapy

The last great triumph of therapeutics, namely chemotherapy, may at first sight seem a departure from this biological approach. But it is not so remote as it appears. Strictly speaking the treatment of any malady by a chemical agent of known composition might be included in the term chemotherapy; actually, however, it is almost universally limited to the treatment of parasitic diseases by chemical control of the infecting agent without marked toxic effects on the patient. Ehrlich's side-chain theory elaborated to explain the formation of antitoxins led him on to the idea of the possibility of a toxin being completely overcome by a drug instead of an antitoxin. An organic compound might carry a strong poison on a side chain which could attach itself to and neutralize a bacterial poison or, still better, thus destroy the microbe itself—a great sterilizing therapy as he called it. Whether his theory holds or not we must admit that it led to the discovery of salvarsan, whereby a much larger dose of arsenic could be given without harm to the host. Yet that a biological reaction enters into this is clear from the fact that salvarsan does not kill protozoa *in vitro*, but only when the cell sets the arsenic free in an ionized pentavalent form. Here then was the beginning of chemotherapy, and the history of its latest and greatest success illustrates some of these considerations very well. Sulphonamide was synthesized in 1908 and used in the preparation of dyes, the fastness of which was found to be much increased thereby. It was thought that this quality was due to the union of this synthetic dye with the protein cells of the wool. Although in 1919 some of such dyes were noted to be bactericidal, no clinical application of this fact was begun until 1930. Five years later prontosil was reported on favourably in the treatment of erysipelas, and Domagk came to the conclusion that it had no bactericidal effect *in vitro* but acted only in living tissues. Colebrook and Kenny reported very favourably on its effects in puerperal sepsis. This led to great interest in the whole group of these drugs, culminating in the preparation of sulphapyridine (M. & B. 693). It is not yet certain how they act, but apparently they bring the chemical processes of the microbe to a standstill, so that it becomes harmless to the cells of the body and can then be devoured by the phagocytes or other defensive agents of the organism.

It is a very interesting fact that just as the body can be educated by small doses of a toxin to resist larger doses, so a microbe can be educated by small doses of these drugs to resist larger doses of them. In the earlier days of salvarsan therapy it was soon found that inadequate doses made the spirochaete resistant to any further doses. The same is true of sulphonamides. This I think proves that in chemotherapy a biological reaction is excited, so that it turns out to be allied to and not remote from the more directly biological methods I spoke of earlier.

Changing Conceptions of Therapeutics

Here we see a definite relationship between the change in the conception of disease and the methods adopted to counter it. As long as the old conception held that disease was something imposed by malign influence from without, magical methods of treatment seemed appropriate. With the new conception that disease is a series of reactions in the body itself to changes in its external or internal environment, it was realized that rational therapeutics must take the form of utilizing and aiding the natural defences of the body. Between those two phases there was of necessity a slow transition from the attribution of magical properties to herbs to the extraction of standardized alkaloids from them.

To look into an old text-book of therapeutics is a chastening experience, for much of it was not merely useless but frequently actually harmful. For a long time this must have been almost unavoidable, since physiology and pathology had not advanced sufficiently to be of real help. But therapeutics has a special difficulty of its own, and that is the almost complete impossibility of rigidly controlled experiment, with consequent doubtful validity in the interpretation of the results. Starling in reproving physiologists for their rather contemptuous attitude towards therapeutics reminded them that they were careful to cut out all complicating factors from their experiments, which the clinician is quite unable to do in dealing with the patient's body as the unit. Moreover, controlled experiments on patients are seldom justifiable. One might mention, as an exception, the controlled experiment of giving alkalis to one side of a scarlet fever ward and not to the other, which led to the conclusion that alkalis diminished the liability to scarlatinal nephritis. But it is a delicate point to decide how soon the evidence is complete enough to make the continuance of the experiment ethically justifiable. There is of course the control by comparing the statistics of the results given by older and newer methods. Judged in this way the success of the sulphonamides was rapidly established. I always maintain that the genuineness of a therapeutical discovery can often be gauged by the way in which its applicability extends. Insulin is a good example of this, since its use has now extended even to the treatment of mental disease, and certainly the sulphonamides are a striking testimony to the truth of this dictum.

With this assertion I must draw my remarks to a close. Living in an age which has discovered more scientific methods of dealing out suffering and death than any preceding epoch, it is a relief to turn to the consideration of the enormous increase in our means of healing. Indeed, we may fairly claim that the last hundred years have seen greater advance in this respect than any other period. For centuries the pool of healing remained stagnant, but in these latter days it has indeed become active, and the future is full of hope for still further developments in the evolution of therapeutics.

It was suggested to me that I might enlarge my title thus: 'From Witchcraft to Chemotherapy and back again', for surely never in recent centuries have horoscopes been so diligently consulted or magical remedies so ardently sought. Unreason always increases in times of national distress. But that is too large a topic to embark upon. Let me end with a note of interrogation: the wisdom of one generation is often the foolishness of the next. What will coming generations think of ours?

Milton Keynes UK
Ingram Content Group UK Ltd.
UKHW041519181024
449640UK00009B/70

9 781107 632455